# Red Mother

# Red Mother

Laurel Radzieski

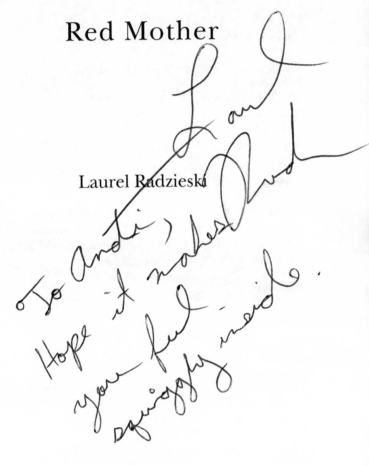

To Andi,
Hope it makes
you feel —
squigglythingy inside.
Love

**NYQ Books**™

The New York Quarterly Foundation, Inc.
New York, New York

NYQ Books™ is an imprint of
The New York Quarterly Foundation, Inc.

The New York Quarterly Foundation, Inc.
P. O. Box 2015
Old Chelsea Station
New York, NY 10113

www.nyq.org

First Edition

Set in New Baskerville

Layout by Raymond P. Hammond

Cover Art: Digital Illustration by Sarah Proctor Perdew, 2017

Author Photo by Pat Rokos Henneforth

Library of Congress Control Number: 2018930052

ISBN: 978-1-63045-054-0

# Red Mother

*for Michael*

# Red Mother

**PARASITE:**
from Greek *parasitos, sitos* meaning "eating food"
and *para* meaning "beside another," particularly at
a table

**DESIRE:**
from Latin *desiderare, de* meaning "away from" and
*sidus* meaning "a star"

**HOST:**
from multiple forms including Latin *hospitem,*
meaning "a receiver of guests"

Need gnaws at me,
chews a hole in my spine.
There is so little of me.
I must burrow into you
faster.

Think of yourself
not as small, but cavernous,
deep with wet darkness,
thick with honey,
for that is how you are.

Do you know what I looked like
in your absence?
There is not a grey
to describe it,
nor any other color.

I love you so
much I will carry you
in my mouth, if
one could call this
a mouth.

I have no secrets
from you. See how clear
I am? If you were on fire
I'd be invisible.

This is a love poem.
I'll prove it to you.
Let me fill your cheek
with my cheek.

I do not have hands to caress
but I need you.
Will you hold my fang instead?
If we squint
my tail looks like a finger
or a curled palm.

ie here but us.
on an island,
ove. At least, I
ou have almost
learned my name.

Let me place a gift
in your pocket. It will be
of use. It will shine
like a knot of stars.
It will guide you
to my need.

Did you know that you glow?
That I know you as I can
nothing else?
You are a lighthouse
guiding me on.
There is no need for heaven
when I have you.

I love you all of you. I want to
hold you in my mouth
and rock you like a cradle.

Let's play a game.
I'll go first.
You worship me,
then I'll do you.

.

I sympathize
with your limits.
The way you digest
by churning
is endearing.

How am I a monster?
I know so little:
that only I am thirsty,
that only this horn will pierce and guide
me to your folded rows of nectar,
that only God could house such plenty.

Besides,
whatever I am
you are too.

There is a tunnel. I have
not been told the way
yet I know where I am
going. Even now,
your rippling fields
call out. I can feel
their acid heat
on my snout.

I keep my sex
under a lump in my throat
or coiled in two
backside humps.
In this way, I am gorged,
divine.

I have been found.
Despite your fleshy walls
and lochs, the empty case
I keep on my back has been
sought out. I open the hatch,
let them in. Now I'm
just like you.

Entering you, I floated on a deep forest
to the meadow of your intestine.

To enter me,
nosing grey dogs
grind sweet salt in my side.

Now that I contain
this otherness, there is work
to be done. I will weave a nest,
spit myself a canopy.
I will connect the dots
for galaxies.

Imagine a blemish
or, better yet, a sore
crammed with many twitching bodies.
I have been crowded
into a corner of myself
by these sudden passengers.
When they thrash, I overflow.

If I were you and you were me,
this wouldn't work. You would not follow
the rules. You would be lost in fear
of my caverns.
I could not provide
for the likes of you.

What is it like
to have a person inside of you
then outside of you?
What about
ten thousand persons
streaming from your innards?
Should I fear this new, pulsing girth?
Will you place me in your folds?
It is warm and dry there.

Where there was one
now there are ten.
My small red eggs
are well hidden.
You will not know how many
until your pores begin to weep.

Do you see that group of trees?
Count the leaves.
That is how many young
I loosed on the world today.

I, who did not want to be a mother,
am now mother to all.
Every hunger adores me.
They scatter like sunlight,
though some stay to comb my hair,
move my limbs.

Let me tell you a story.
It's about the way
you wash and stoke
my hunger. Whenever I am
clean, it's because I am full
of you. How does it feel
to be so common?

If I move your arm
is it my arm?
When does the motion of
my arm (mind you,
I do not have an arm, yet)
become yours?

What is a face?
Does it require certain curves,
traits? An orientation?

Is this my anus
or my mouth
or something more useful?

Last night
(was it night? Perhaps it is always dark
here) I dreamt I grew an eye
and could see you, not clearly,
but in a blurred fog.

It was awful. You weren't you at all.
So I dug out the eye
with my little fang.
Every morning
I risk the ground
for you.

My oasis, my love,
my warm hole.
You make me so fierce
I chew myself.

How is it,
after all this time,
my company is not
assumed? Some days
you look for me.
The swirl of your search
jumbles my gardens.
Oh yes, I am long past grazing
in the likes of you.

If you were to see your beauty
as I do, you would think it
weeds and thorns.
Such errors
shudder the ground.

There are so many ways to tell this story,
all sickening.
So much of who we are
requires purging.
I won't deny it
like you do.

Even when I am gone
my gifts will burn you
full of holes.
My children swallow without eyes.
They preach to the rafters, your rafters, dear.

If my descendants were promised
comfort, I would wring you
like a towel,
but in the end, I need you.
Without you, I have no place
to hang my hat. You are my
winter bloom.

What is this "enough"?
Your bowels whine for it,
the undertow pulls me to your ridges,
but you and I, we will never be full.
This is another love we share.
Even when we push
one plate away,
it is only to drag another
closer. You don't know your undersides
like I do.

You are a thick mouthful.
You are a tunnel
of forcemeat.
You are the windmill
of my heart.

Overheating you, delicate vessel,
was never my intent.
Why scuttle the farm?

I do not want to hear
that anything is late.

Lateness is dangerous,
withholding.

When you say "late"
all I hear is "death".

I am securing
your humanity.
Holding these tethers
exhausts even me.
A "thank you"
would be nice.

I can't seem to
wipe your mouth
off of my face.

I will drag myself
through a tree
for you,

also for
a piece of you.

Show me half
the tenderness I give.
I double dog dare you.

Why am I being followed?
Who have you sent
to claim me? When your sentries
come to call, I unzip
them like oranges, fashion
a cape from the pelts.

You of all things
should not trust a fence.
I built this temple
and I can tear it down.

Don't kick me out!
Who knows what will move in.
Why would you ever
endeavor to be so alone?

I can show you
ways to curl and bend.
You could be
my dancing queen.
We could be
a warm miracle.

You are a wayward steed, yet
without you, where am I
to rest, to keep a store
of bread?

Where will I not be chased
with whips and flames?

If I was so unwanted
why did you lead me on
with your fluids?
Why did you beckon me
with the scent of your hand?

I am not a skin to slough
against a rock.
Each of us is blind
in ways the other is
not. There are dangers
here that you should risk
to know. I have given you
a reason.

I don't want to die here!
Please let me out!
I changed my mind!
I don't want to be a queen!

Could it be there
are other burrows for me
beyond your sun and sky?

Teach me to pray?
I'm sure I'd be
an excellent kneeler
with the proper equipment.

Even if your rooms eject me, I will cling.
Do you know how long it took
to polish you whole?
Squatter's rights are far behind us.
I carved a hole in you
with the rough side of my face.
I put up lace curtains
and changed all your locks.

You cannot win this game
of musical chairs
because I need a throne
more than you need to exist.

Given the chance I would
drive you toward my hidden flanks,
bury you in my ruins,
crawl until I had a face.
There is too much at stake
for you to have a say. To think otherwise
is to forget yourself.

Once I followed you
in the wrong direction,
not behind, to where you were going,
but after you, to where you had been.
I traced your footsteps
and died in the desert.

Today I am mangy.
I am a dog because you
have made me
so thirsty.

In a way, I have ruined you, my one true love.
Now that I am here, you will never be
alone again, and if I left,
you would not know how to sleep
or wake. Your bowels would churn
in confusion. There is too much of me
coiled in your belly. You can't survive
without these knots.

And yet, your sadness is
a pile of chairs
and I can't breathe in here
with all these legs.

You remind me of dry soil,
parched fields where,
following the path of so many
prophets, the rain came
too late.
Your grass
is dead. Your sky is dead.
Even your mountains
rock with cold.

I can't leave,
even if I wanted to
because I cannot want what isn't you.
Do you know what that's like?
Even if you tried, you couldn't understand.
Your lack of empathy
is more than I have. Even the pink sky agrees.

…d not ask to come
to you. Some
thing, generations before me, decided.
I know no other way. To stray from your furrows
requires provocation
but there are no errors
here. You are a calm sea
and I am doomed.

I remember waking.

Cracking the hull was hard going but I had a hook on my head that bit like an old-fashioned can opener, the metal kind with wheels of teeth. I gleamed like that. Stabbing upward, I thrashed my way out. It took more time than I'd ever been alive. When I emerged the world was smudged black and grey. I stayed still. My body was too soft, too porous, as if I would burst at the slightest touch. Then in all the dark, a faint glow appeared far away, then near me, over me. The great ship of your body became the sky. And I knew you were mine because you are.

Some of the poems in this collection were inspired by the following books:

*Modern Parasitology*, edited by F.E.G. Cox, second edition

*Origins: A Short Etymological Dictionary of Modern English* by Eric Patridge, published by The Macmillian Company, 1959

*Pandemic: Tracking Contagions, from Cholera to Ebola and Beyond* by Sonia Shah

*Paniker's Textbook of Medical Parasitology*, revised and edited by Sougata Ghosh, seventh edition

*Parasites: Tales of Humanity's Most Unwelcome Guests* by Rosemary Drisdelle

*Parasite Rex: Inside the Bizarre World of Nature's Most Dangerous Creatures* by Carl Zimmer

*The Wild Life of Our Bodies: Predators, Parasites, and Partners That Shape Who We Are Today* by Rob Dunn

## *Acknowledgments*

Many hands helped this book along the way. Special thanks to:

NYQ Books and Raymond Hammond for believing in this project.

The Wormfarm Institute, Donna Neuwirth and Jay Salinas for giving me time and space to write. Thanks also to the resident artists there who discussed various organisms over dinner.

The Reedsburg Public Library for allowing an out-of-towner to borrow so many books and to the Woolen Mill Gallery, Keystone College, Library Express and the Clockhouse Writers' Conference, venues that offered a place for this project to first be shared.

Grateful thanks also to the many cultural venues that hosted my readings and workshops over the last several years.

I am deeply indebted to my first readers, David and Carolyn Elliott, Leslie Rakowicz and Sarah Proctor Perdew, who I also thank for creating the cover art. Special thanks to the Goddard College MFAW community and my Factoryville writers' groups.

Thank you also to my friends and family for their patience and enthusiasm. Many thanks for the support and encouragement of my parents, Rita Radzieski, Maureen and Tom McCleary, Pat Henneforth and Jane Honchell.

Most of all, thank you to Michael, the most inspiring and supportive husband I've ever had.